The Mediterranean Diet Cookbook for Beginners

The Complete Guide Quick & Easy Recipes to build healthy habits.

DESSERTS

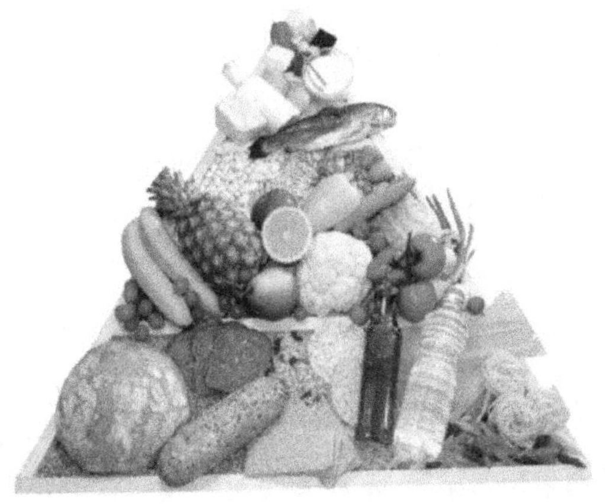

OLIVIA BROWN

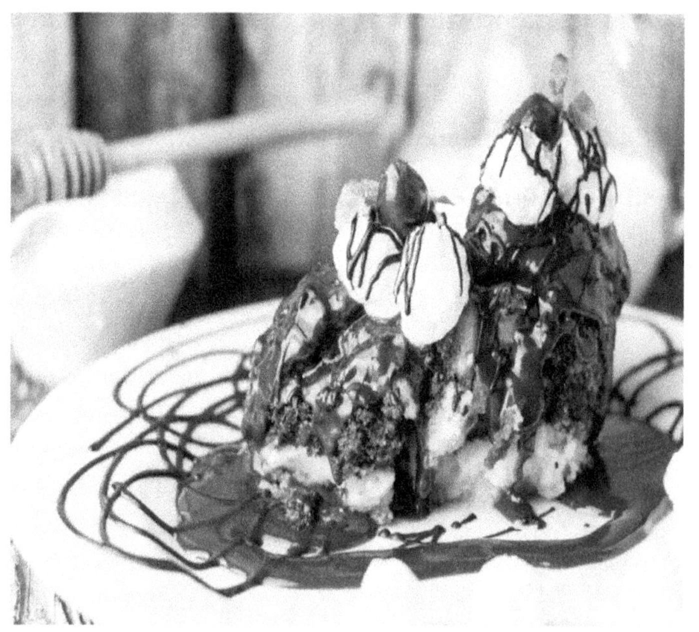

1. Greek Kourambiedes

Total Time: 30 minutes

Difficulty Level: low

Servings: 3 dozen

Ingredients:

- 2 cups of all-purpose flour sifted

- 36 whole cloves

- 1 cup of butter unsalted

- Four tablespoons of confectioners' sugar

- One teaspoon of vanilla extract

- 1/2 cup of confectioners' sugar

- 1 cup of chopped pecans

Instructions:

Preheat the oven to 350°F.

In a medium-sized mixing dish, combine the confectioner's sugar and the butter. Combine extract of vanilla, flour and pecans.

Make balls of walnut size and add each of the cloves in the balls. Put in the preheated oven for about 15-18 minutes on a cookie sheet. Roll them in powdered sugar while the cookies are still warm. Take away the cloves. Serve.

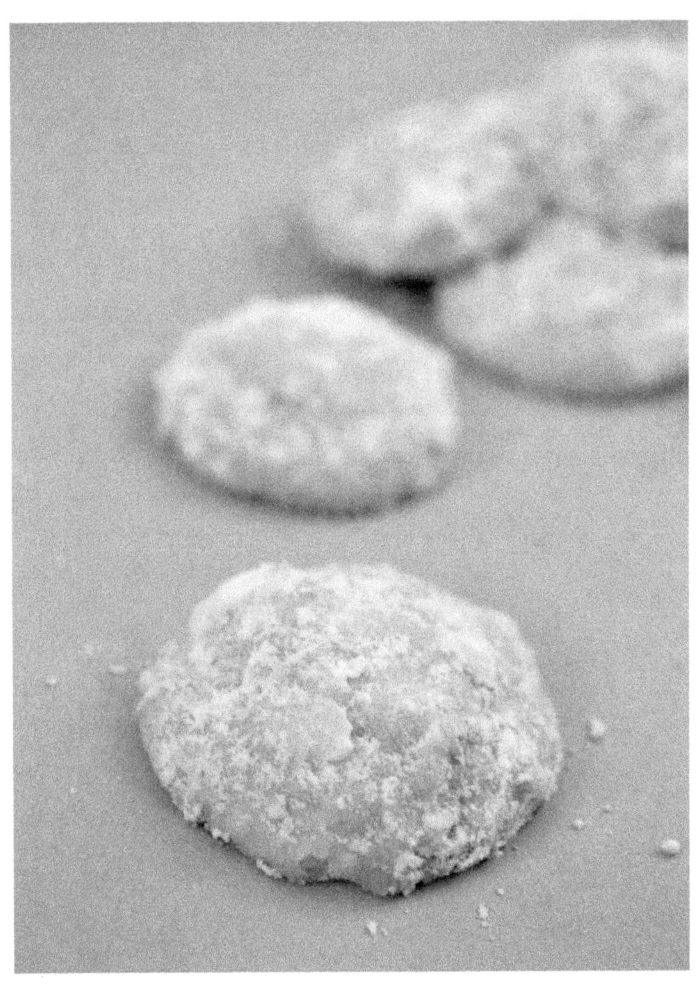

Total Time: 25 minutes

Difficulty Level: low

Servings: 4

Ingredients:

- *1 cup of light whipped cream*

- *1/2 cup of Thompson raisins*

- *Four tablespoons of Kahlua, divided*

- *1/2 cup of sugar*

- *3 cups of Greek Yogurt fat-free*

- *One teaspoon of vanilla extract*

- *1/2 cup of roughly chopped hazelnuts, shelled*

- *1/2 cup of roughly chopped pistachios, shelled*

- *One teaspoon of cinnamon*

Instructions:

In a small microwave-safe dish, combine raisins with two teaspoons of Kahlua rum. 50 seconds high microwave. Return to the microwave again after stirring for another 30 seconds. Raisins are going to absorb Kahlua and get delicious and plump. Put them aside.

In a food processor, add pistachios and hazelnuts to chop them coarsely.

In a large mixing bowl with a hand, combine the Greek yogurt, whipped cream, two kahlua tablespoons, vanilla extract, sugar, and cinnamon.

You ought to cover the yogurt mix for an hour or until you are ready to assemble at this step.

To make it perfect, begin with pouring into the base of the serving glass with the yogurt mixture.

Place the Kahlua and the mixed nuts on top.

Top up the yogurt mixture with nut sprinkling.

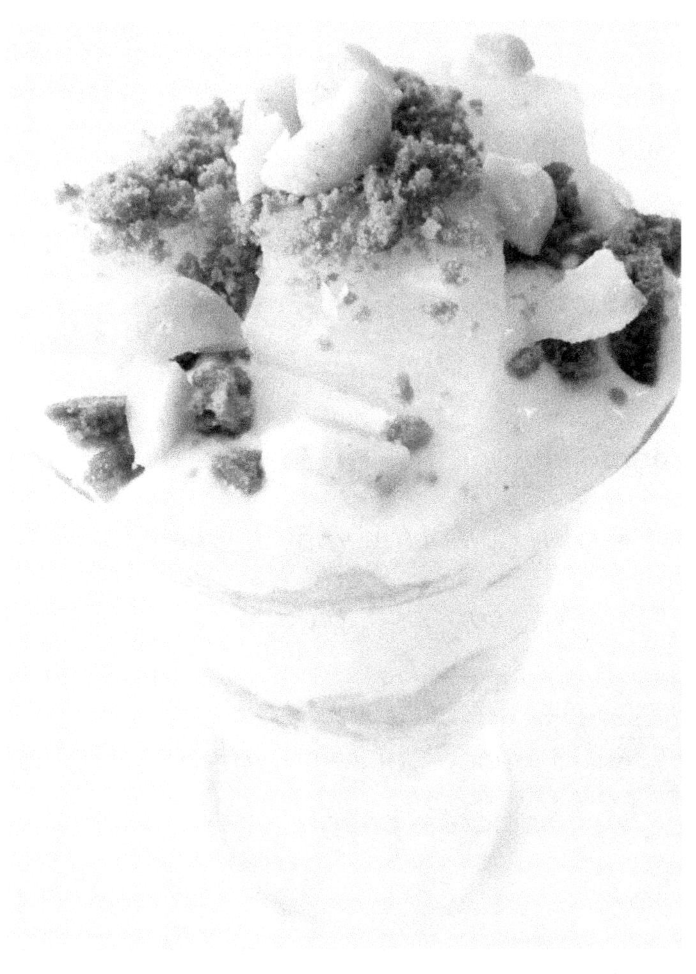

Total Time: 30 minutes

Difficulty Level: low

Servings: 2 dozen

Ingredients:

- *Half cup of the vanilla/ white chips*

- *Half cup of thoroughly macadamia nuts, chopped*

- *18 ounces of refrigerated chocolate chip cookie dough*

Instructions:

Preheat the oven to 350°F.

Combine the dough, nuts and chips in a large mixing dish. Use your hands until everything is mixed together well. Divide and set aside the dough into two equal portions.

Bake in the oven for 12 to 15 minutes until light brown.

Divide it into 1-inch slices. Bake 4 to 5 minutes longer. Allow biscotti before serving to cool down fully.

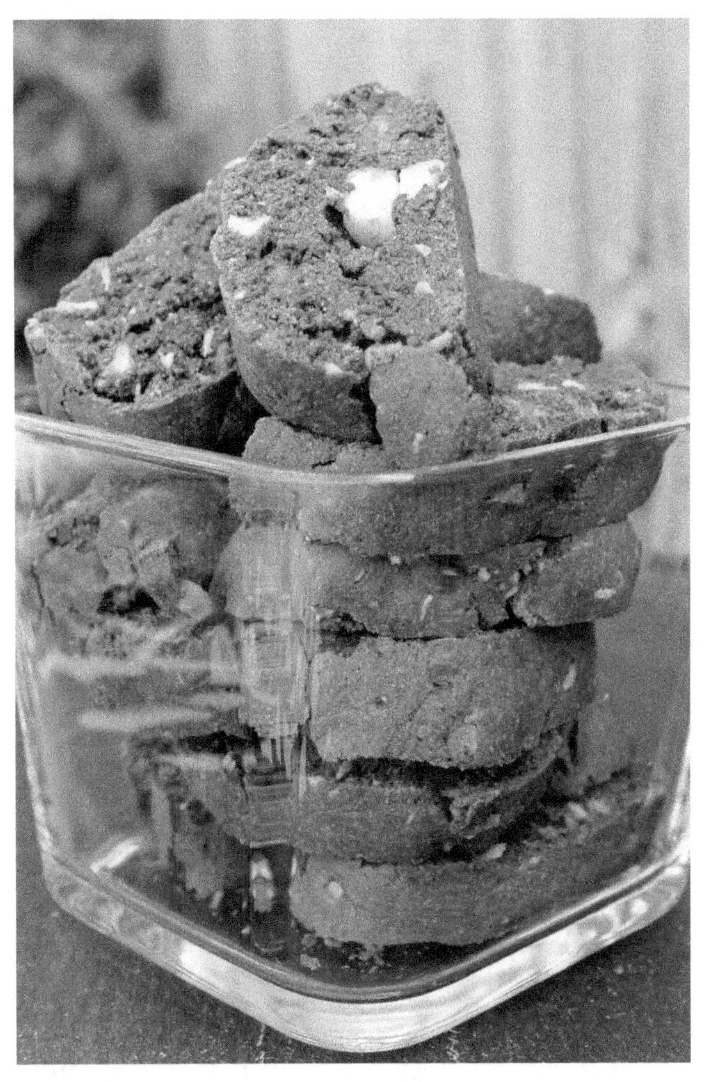

Total Time: 17 minutes

Difficulty Level: low

Servings: 2

Ingredients

- Egg white, 1

- Lemon juice, one teaspoon

- Water, 3 cups

- Castor sugar, 50 g

Instructions

Heat water, sugar and lemon juice within a casserole until the temperature reach 243°F. In the meantime, whisk the white eggs to produce soft peaks.

Add to the egg Whites and continue blending when the mixture of water, sugar and lemon juice reaches 243° F. Mix until room temperature is reached.

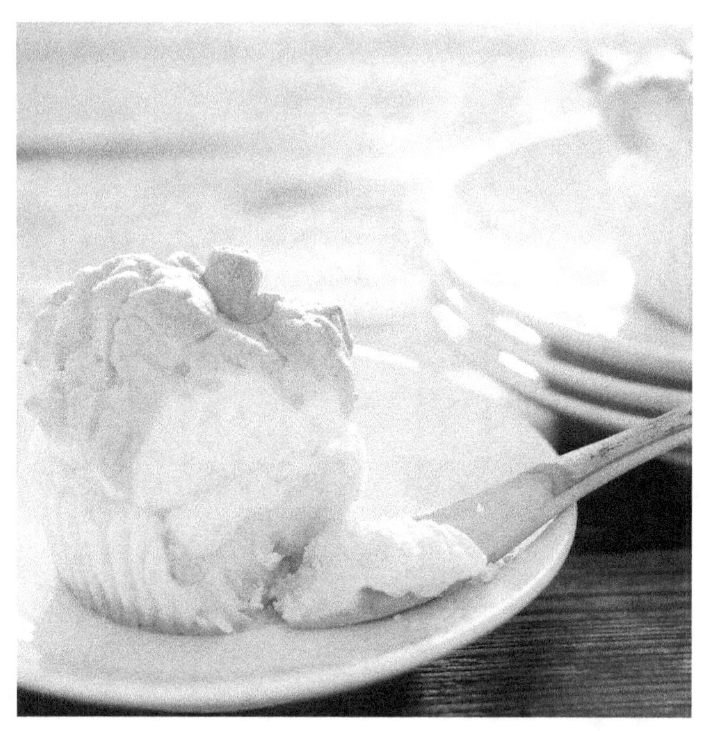

5. Delicious Pumpkin Pie Muffins

Total Time: 30 minutes

Difficulty Level: low

Servings: 12

Ingredients:

- 1/2 cup of brown sugar packed

- 15 ounces of pumpkin puree

- 1/4 teaspoon of baking soda

- 1/4 teaspoon of baking powder

- 10 ounces of low-fat milk

- 1/2 cup of flour

- 1/2 teaspoon of salt

- Whipped cream for serving

- 1/4 cup of white sugar

- Two large-sized eggs

- 1 1/2 teaspoons of pumpkin pie spice

Instructions:

Preheat the oven to 350°F. Grate a muffin bowl with oil.

Mix the breadcrumbs, meal, salt, and bread powder in a small basin.

Combine white sugar, eggs, spices, brown sugar, pumpkin puree and fatty milk in a medium-size mixing bowl. In a large blender, combine the dry ingredients. Split the batter between the muffin cups equally.

In a preheated convection oven, cook for 24 to 25 minutes. Refrigerate for 10 minutes.

Refrigerate the muffins after removing them from the pot for at least 3 hours or overnight. Serve on top of the muffins with whipped cream.

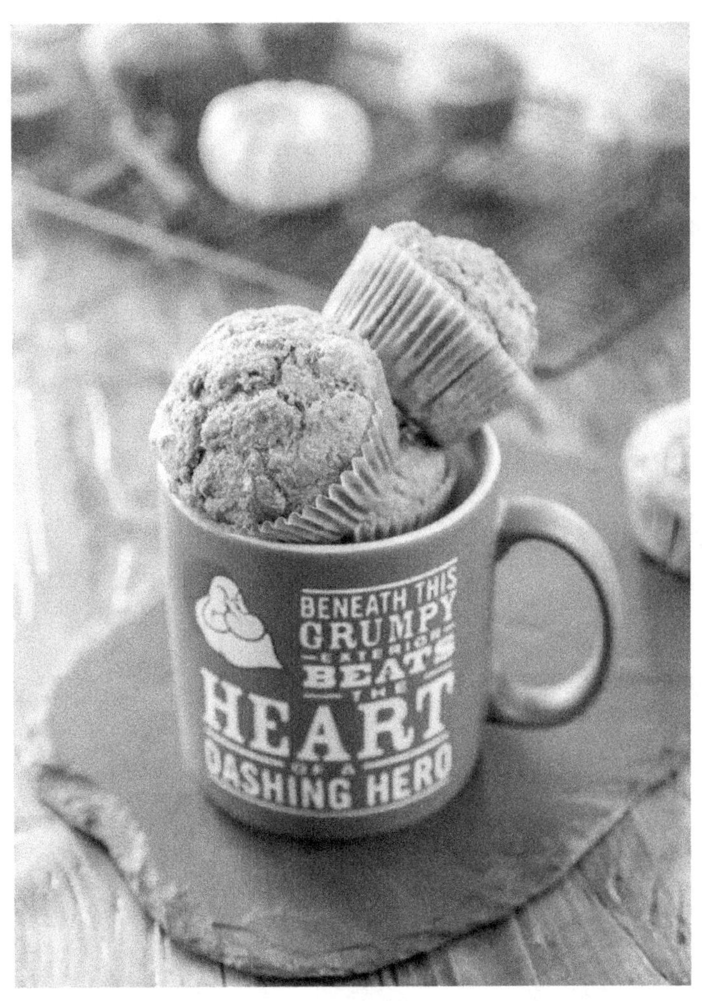

BENEATH THIS
GRUMPY
BEATS
THE
HEART
DASHING HERO

Total Time: 1 hour 15 minutes

Difficulty Level: low

Servings: 8

Ingredients

- Fresh butter, 1 cup

- Eggs, 6

- Sugar, 1 cup

- Zest of 1 lemon

- Milk, 1 cup

- Flour, 2 cups

- Fine semolina, 1 cup

- Sugar, 4 cups

- Baking powder, two teaspoons

- Water, 3 cups

Ingredients for the ice cream:

- Juice from 2 lemons

- Vanilla flavored ice cream, 1 kg

- Sugar, 100 grams

- Saffron, one dose

Instructions

To 225F, prepare an oven. Mix the butter and sugar inside a mix, then combine in the eggs and thoroughly beat the combination; last, add all the other ingredients and then mix again till the mixture is fluffy. Now place the mixture in a mound and bake it for 10–12 minutes or until fully done inside the oven.

After the cake has been baked, remove it from the oven and cool, then cut into four to six equal pieces.

Heat a pan over medium heat and add a few drops of the lemon juice and saffron to it, then pour it over the entire ice cream after cooling.

Put an ice cream scoop over pieces of cake and serve.

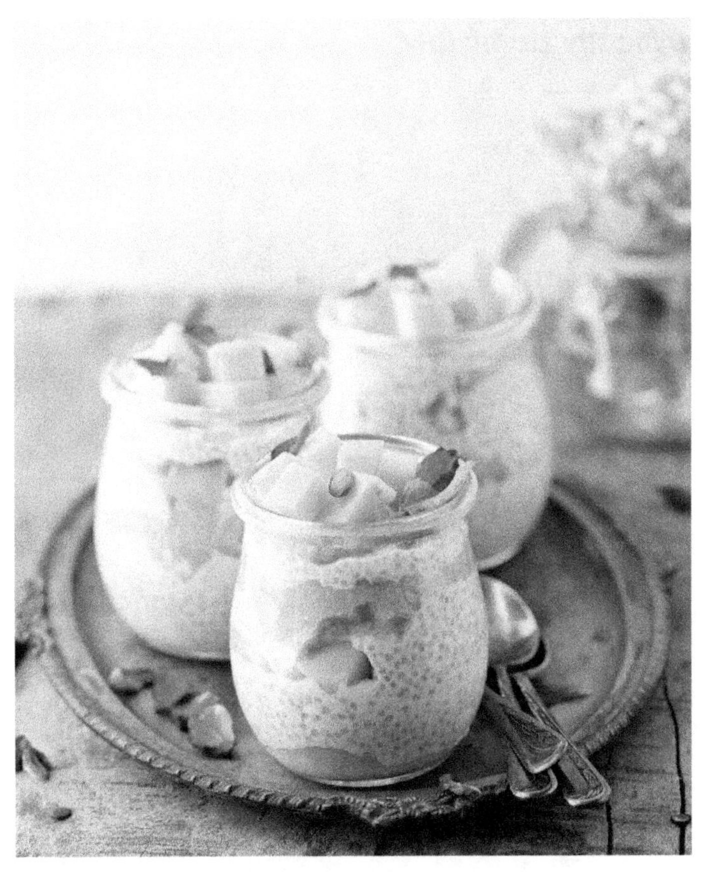

Total Time: 30 minutes

Difficulty Level: low

Servings: 4

Ingredients:

- Two tablespoons of good fig jam

- 4 to 5 oz. of goat cheese

- One sheet of puff pastry, store-bought

- 1/4 cup of roughly chopped fresh mint leaves

- 1/4 cup of roughly chopped walnuts

- 8 oz. of fresh black mission figs

- One tablespoon of butter melted

Instructions:

Preheat the oven to 375°F.

Place a parchment paper-lined bakery with thawed puff pastry and cut in four rectangular slices.

Spread goat cheese on every slice. Then add the jam, figs and chopped walnuts.

Brush the figs and sides of the pulp with melted butter.

Turn up somewhat the pastry edges.

Bake the pastry in a golden and puffy crust for 18-20 minutes.

Garnish with chopped mint leaves and extra walnuts if preferred.

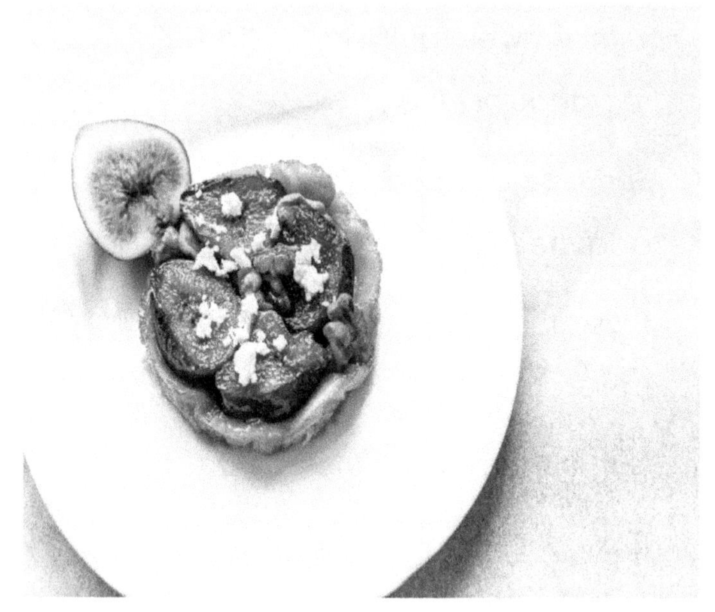

Total Time: 45 minutes

Difficulty Level: low

Servings: 4

Ingredients

- Organic eggs, 4

- Extra-virgin olive oil, 75ml

- Sugar, 100g

- Organic natural yogurt, 125g

- wheat flour, 100g

- Based yogurt, half cup

- Organic flour, 70g

- Baking powder, two teaspoons

- sea salt, one pinch

Instructions

Preheat the oven to 160F approximately. Turn the batter to a nice cooking consistency and mix up all the components together very well.

Pour in a lightly greased batter with olive oil and bake in the oven for approximately 10-12 minutes or until thoroughly done.

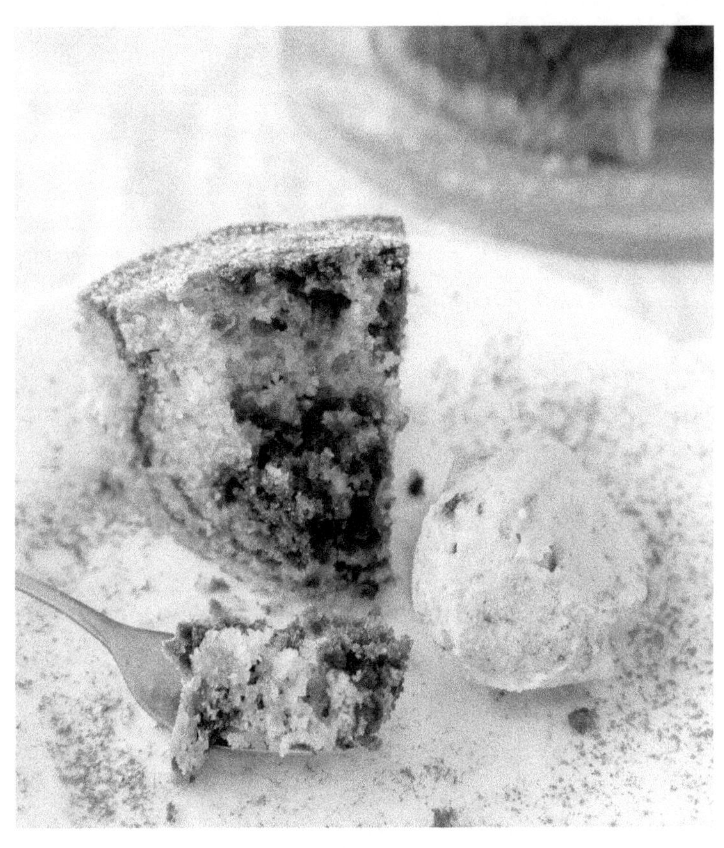

34

Total Time: 30 minutes

Difficulty Level: low

Servings: 6

Ingredients:

- Four tablespoons of white sugar

- One teaspoon of vanilla extract

- 2 cups of water

- 1/2 cup of whole milk

- 1/2 cup of short-grain white rice uncooked

- Four tablespoons of cornstarch

- 1/4 teaspoon of ground cinnamon

- 2 cups of whole milk

Instructions:

Bring rice and water to a boil in a casserole. Turn the flame down immediately to medium-low. Cook, uncover, gentle for about 20 minutes until all the water is absorbed.

Raise heat high and add sugar and 2 cups of milk to the bowl.

Combine maize and a quarter of a cup of milk in a separate bowl.

Add the extract of vanilla and maize starch, mix once the mixture has gotten boiling. Take the pot out of the flame.

Sprinkle cinnamon in individual bowls on top of the rice pudding. Allow cooling before serving.

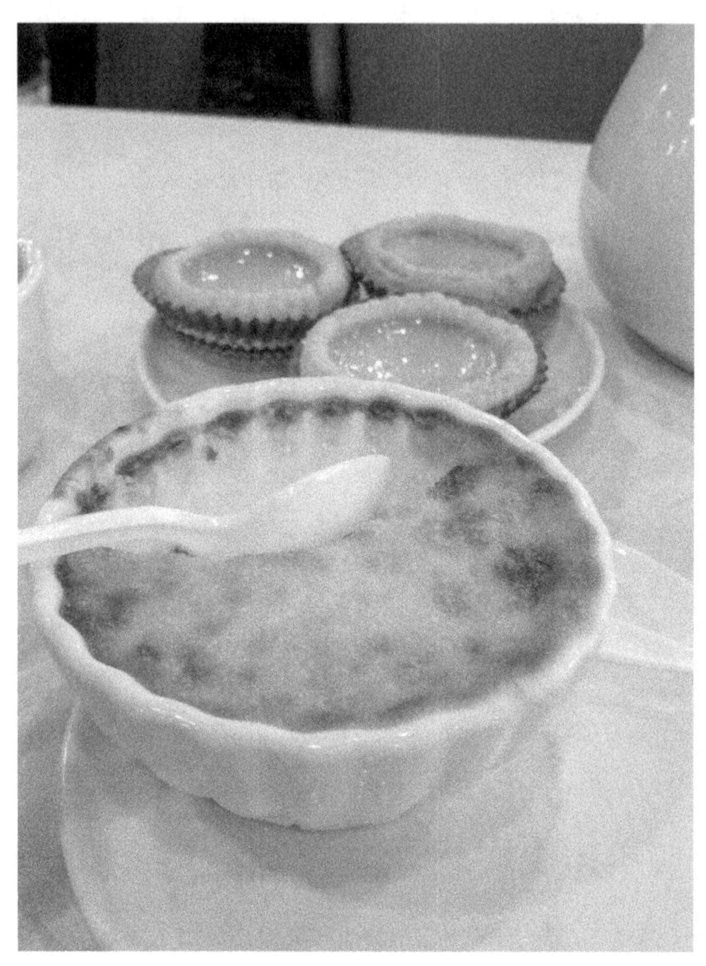

Total Time: 30 minutes

Difficulty Level: low

Servings: 2

Ingredients

- Rolled oats, ¼ cup

- Spelled flour, 1 ½ cups

- Baking powder, 2 ½ teaspoons

- Cinnamon, ½ teaspoon

- Sea salt, ½ teaspoon

- Egg, 1

- Orange juice ⅓ cup

- Olive oil, ⅓ cup

- Unsweetened almond milk, ⅓ cup

- Vanilla powder, ½ teaspoon

- Maple syrup, ⅓ cup

- Orange zest, ½ tablespoon

- Chopped almonds, ¼ cup

- Grated carrot, 1

Instructions

Preheat the oven to 350oF approximately. Inside the muffin cups, brush some oil. Now add some salt into the bowl to your flour, oats and baking powder. Add olive oil, orange and almond milk eggs, and blend with a few drops of vanilla essence and maple syrups.

Mix these ingredients properly. When the batter is ready, place this blend in the muffins and bake for 12-15 minutes at 375F. Take the muffins from the oven after cooking and rest for a while before serving.

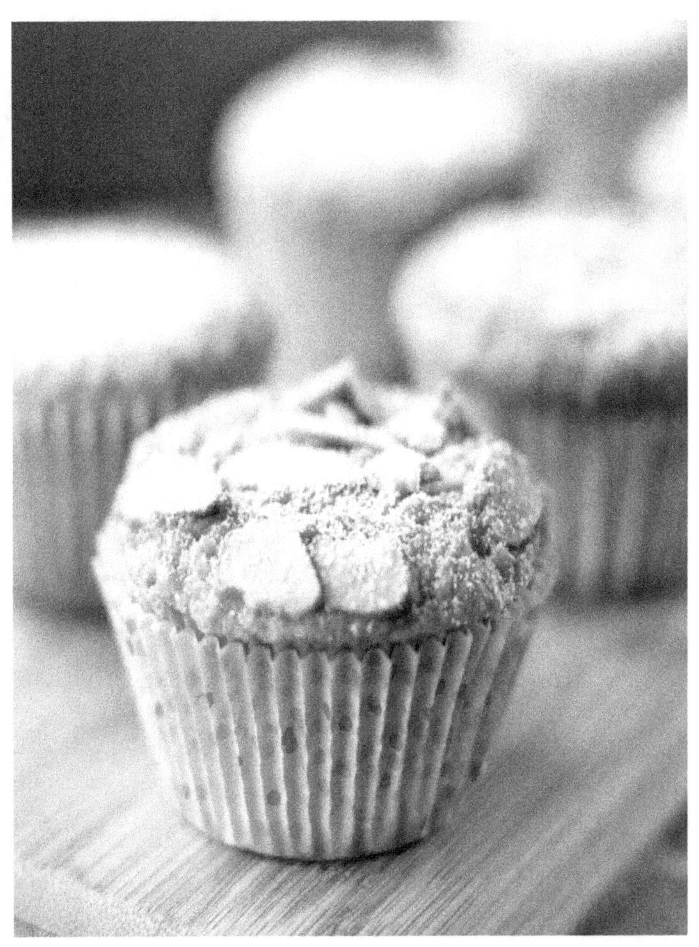

11. Butter Pecan Crispy Cookies

Total Time: 30 minutes

Difficulty Level: low

Servings: 4

Ingredients:

- 1/2 teaspoon of salt

- 1 1/2 cups of halves pecan

- 2 cups of all-purpose flour

- 2/3 cup of brown sugar packed

- 1 cup of butter softened

- One medium-sized egg

Instructions:

Preheat the oven to 350°F.

Mix the egg, brown sugar and softened butter together in a large mixing dish. Mix until fully combined.

Gradually add salt and flour to the mixture. Cool for at least one hour, covered.

Roll in pieces of the dough and roll them into balls. Arrange two centimetres apart on a baking tray. Press your hands to flatten the balls. Put a nut on a cookie and tap it gently.

Bake about 10 to 15 minutes or until light brown/golden around the edges in a preheated oven.

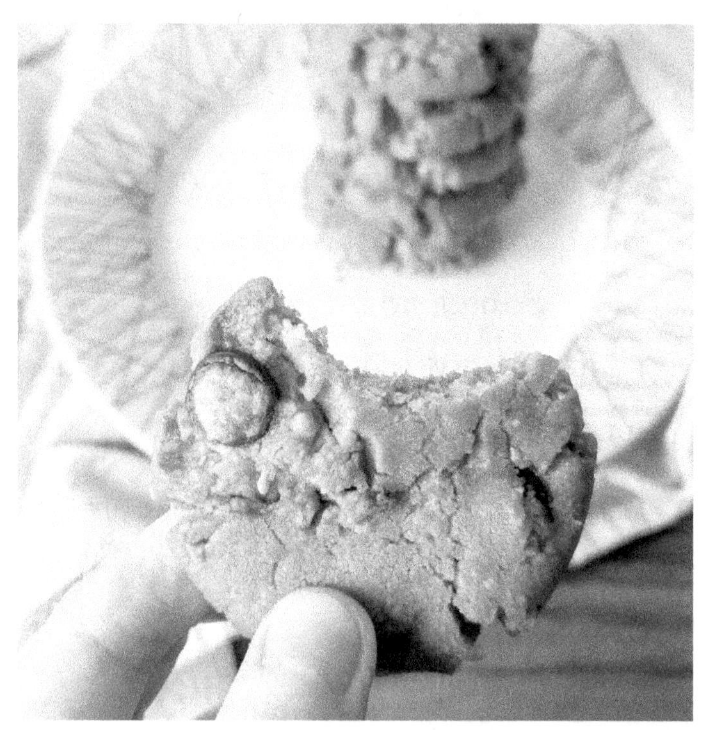

Total Time: 10 minutes

Difficulty Level: low

Servings: 2

Ingredients

- Cashew nuts, 2 cups

- Unsweetened coconut, 1/3 cup

- Dried apricots, 1 cup

- Chopped dates, 1/4 cup

- Lemon zest, one teaspoon

- Orange zest, one teaspoon

- Cinnamon, 1/2 teaspoon

- Salt, 1/8 teaspoon

- Ground ginger, 1/2 teaspoon

Instructions

Combine the cassava noodle with cocoa and apricots. Now add the dates to a food processor. Pulse your components until they are well combined. Add some citrus fruit and spices to the mixture, along with salt. Pulse the components finally to integrate everything well.

Turn dough from your ingredients into small balls and then transform the mixture. You can use it or store it in the refrigerator immediately.

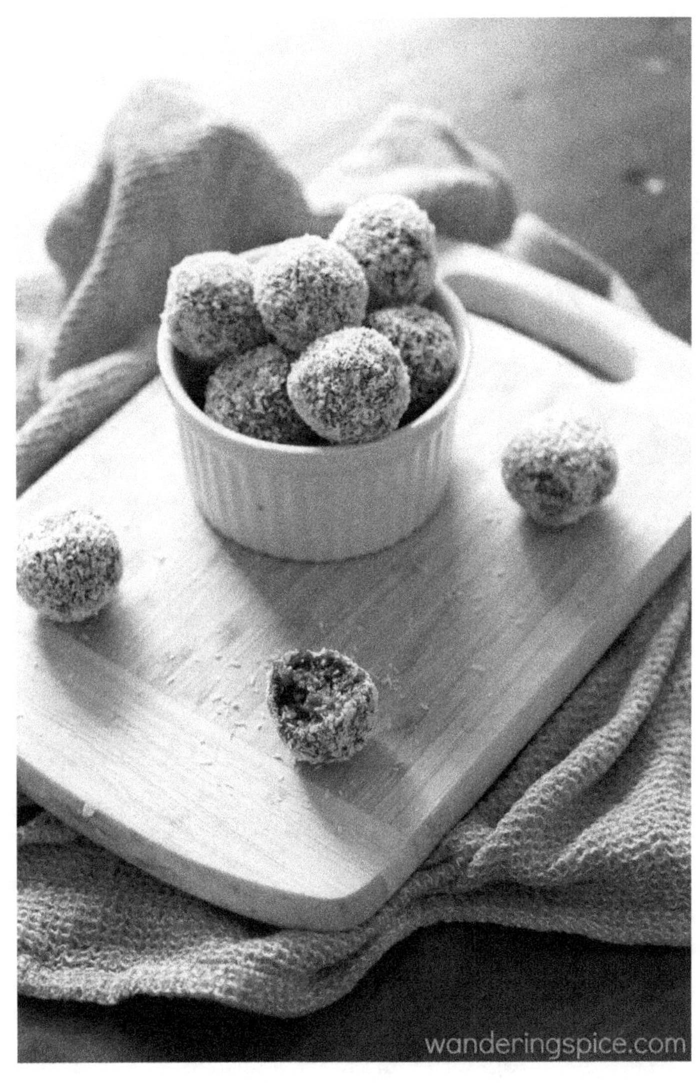

wanderingspice.com

Total Time: 30 minutes

Difficulty Level: low

Servings: 15

Ingredients:

- Ten tablespoons of butter, room temperature

- 1/2 cup+2 tbsp of the powdered sugar

- 1 1/4 cups of flour

- 1/4 teaspoon of salt

For the lemon filling:

- 1/3 cup of fresh lemon juice

- One tablespoon of lemon zest

- Three eggs large-sized at room temperature

- *1 cup of granulated sugar*

- *Three tablespoons of flour*

- *1/2 teaspoon of baking powder*

Instructions:

Preheat the oven to 350°F.

In a mixing dish, combine the polished sugar, salt and flour. Transfer the mixture to a baking tray and squeeze it to produce a crust.

Bake the crust till lightly browned for 15 minutes in a preheated oven.

Combine all the filling elements in a mixing bowl, and beat until creamy and thick.

Spread over the cooked crust uniformly and bake in the oven for another 10 minutes.

Cool the bars fully, dust with powdered sugar and cut into bars.

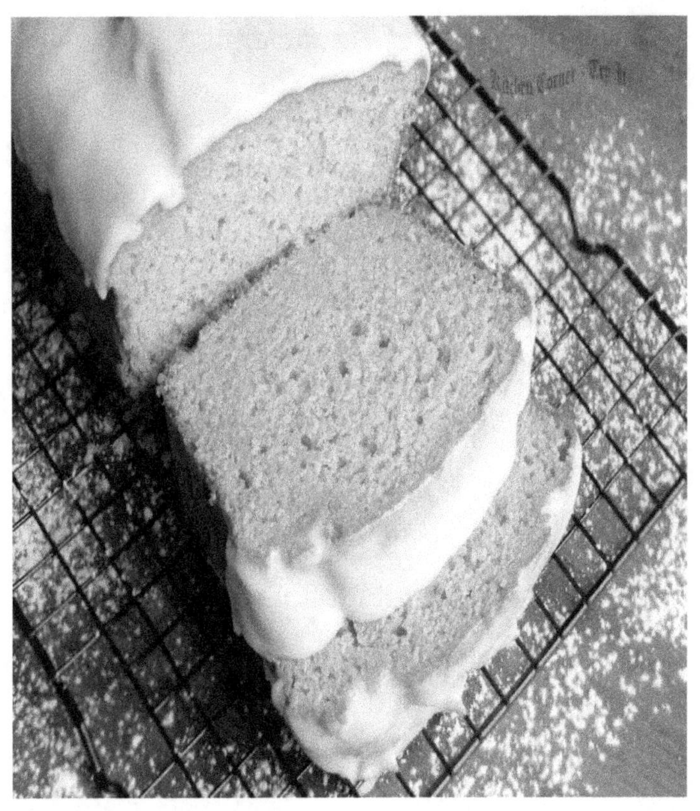

Total Time: 35 minutes

Difficulty Level: low

Servings: 6

Ingredients

- Almond hazelnut flour, 1 cup

- Flour, five tablespoons

- Sugar, 3/4 cup

- Generous pinch of salt

- Vanilla almond extract, 1/2 teaspoon

- Large egg whites, 4

- Brown butter, 2 1/2 ounces

Instructions

Preheat the oven to approximately 375F and line the bottoms of muffin tins

with butter. In a medium-size mixing cup, combine the almonds, hazelnut powder, sugar, and starch, followed by the salt. Combine egg whites, vanilla extract, and browned butter in a separate bowl.

Fill mini muffin tray to the brim with batter. Bake for approximately 12-15 minutes, or until the tops are golden brown. Allow some time for cooling before serving.

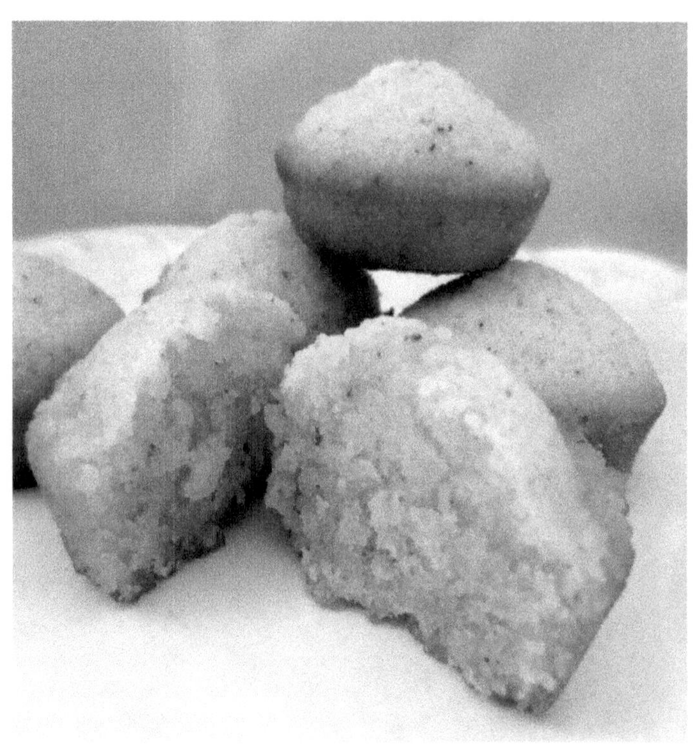

Total Time: 30 minutes

Difficulty Level: low

Servings: 9

Ingredients:

- 1 cup of rolled oats

- 1/2 cup of milk

- One teaspoon of baking soda

- 3/4 cup of peanut butter

- 1 cup of all-purpose flour

- 1/2 teaspoon of salt

- 1/2 cup of brown sugar

- 1/3 cup of chocolate chips

- One teaspoon of vanilla

Instructions:

Preheat oven to 325°F.

Combine the rolled oats, peanut butter, and brown sugar in a mixer until smooth. Combine the milk and vanilla and rolled oats in a separate bowl until well combined.

Combine salt, flour, and baking soda in a small mixing basin, followed by the prepared mixture. Incorporate the chocolate chips.

Spread the mixture evenly into a prepared 8x8-inch baking sheet and bake for 18 to 20 minutes.

Reduce the temperature of the bar somewhat before slicing it.

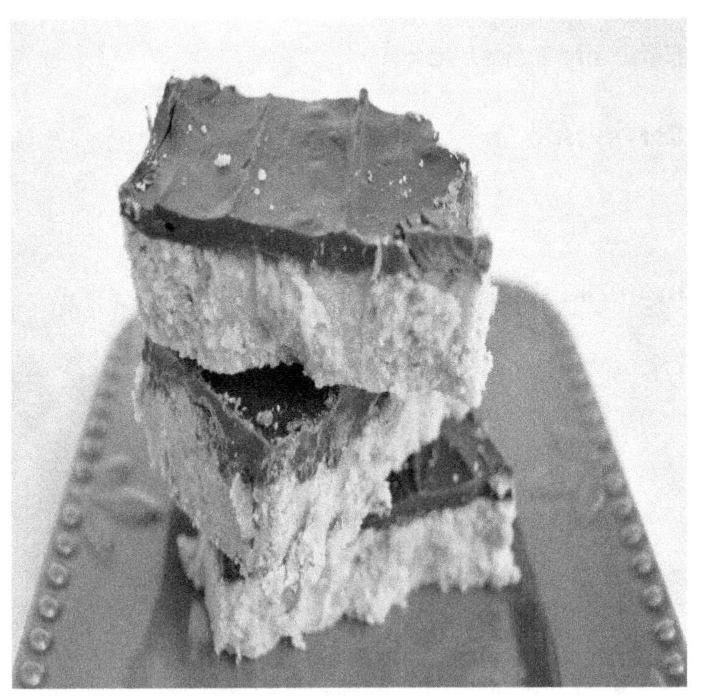

Total Time: 15 minutes

Difficulty Level: low

Servings: 6

Ingredients

- *Sugar, 3 cups*

- *almond extract, one tablespoon*

- *Rosewater, ½ cup*

- *Almonds, 6 cups*

- *Powdered sugar*

Instructions

In a blender, grind the peeled almonds into a powder; this will create the dough. Now add the sugar and almond essence and knead the dough with some rose water.

Once the dough is prepared, roll it into little balls or any other form you choose, cook for a few minutes in a skillet with a little olive oil, and cool to room temperature. Take pleasure in this Greek recipe.

17. Greek Yogurt with Walnuts and Honey

Total Time: 18 minutes

Difficulty Level: low

Servings: 2

Ingredients:

- Cinnamon powder to taste

- Strained Greek yogurt, two and a half cups

- Walnuts, 1 cup

- Vanilla extract, 3/4 teaspoon

- Honey, ½ cup

Instructions:

To begin, whisk together all of the yogurt, honey, and toasted walnuts. Now

 preheat the oven to approximately 180F.

Now toast your walnuts in a single layer, spread them out on a baking sheet, and bake for approximately 8-10 minutes, or until brown and fragrant. Following that, throw the toasted walnuts in a mixing cup and add the honey. Toss one more to coat the walnuts with honey.

Meanwhile, combine the Greek yogurt and vanilla extract in a large mixing basin and divide evenly into 7-8 bowls. Before serving, top the yogurt with walnuts and cinnamon powder and store it in the refrigerator.

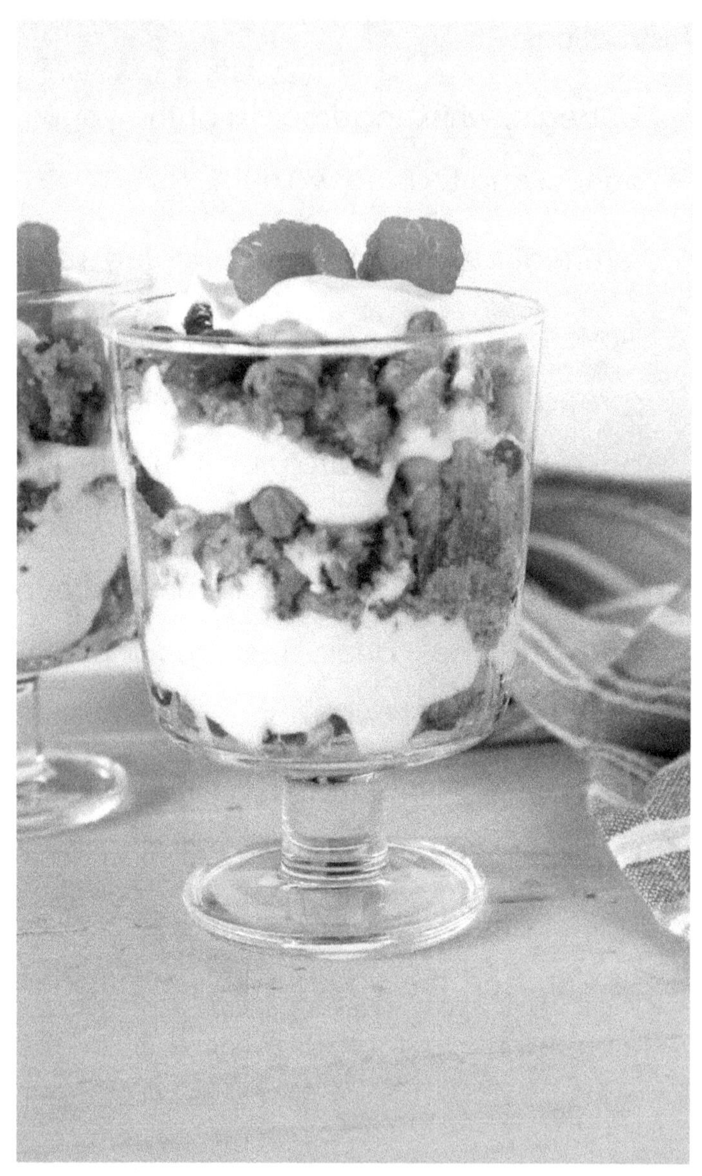

Total Time: 20 minutes

Difficulty Level: low

Servings: 8

Ingredients:

- 1 1/2 teaspoon of coconut extract

- 1 cup of walnut halves

- 3 to 4 tablespoons of honey

- 1 cup of pistachios finely chopped

- 1 1/2 cups of all-purpose flour

- Two sticks of unsalted butter, slice into chunks

- 26 large pitted soft Medjool dates

Instructions:

Expand the Medjool dates partially and stuff each one with a walnut quarter. Close the dates firmly to cover the walnut halves thoroughly.

In the bottom of a small oiled container, place the walnut-stuffed dates.

In a small non-stick skillet over medium-low heat, melt the honey and butter. After adding the coconut extract, stir in the flour. For approximately 5 minutes, or until the flour turns golden brown, stirring regularly.

Fill any gaps in the dates with the flour and honey mixture, evenly dispersed on top. Allow the mixture to solidify before gently pushing the chopped pistachios into the mixture with your hand.

Using a sharp knife, cut the date cake into nine little bars.

For optimal effectiveness, refrigerate the bars for approximately 1 hour or until ready to consume; remove from the refrigerator 10 minutes before serving.

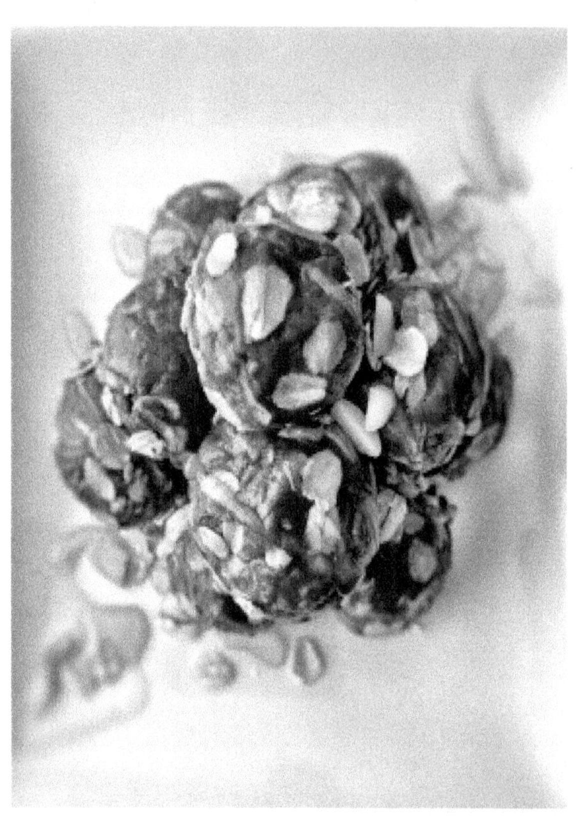

Total Time: 25 minutes

Difficulty Level: low

Servings: 4

Ingredients

- Packed brown sugar, ¼ cup

- Cardamom, 2

- Fresh fruit pears, 6 cups

- Ground cardamom, ½ teaspoon

- Butter melted, three tablespoons

Instructions:

Preheat oven to 450°F. In a small bowl, combine the brown sugar and cardamom. Preheat oven to 350°F. Line a 15x10-inch pan with parchment paper.

Now, evenly distribute the fruit in the prepared pan. Drizzle the butter over the top and sprinkle with the sugar mixture.

Cook for 12 to 15 minutes, uncovered, or when the fruit is soft and starting to tan. Allow for minor cooling.

Now, if desired, sprinkle the Crisp Oats over the ricotta, yogurt, or oatmeal.

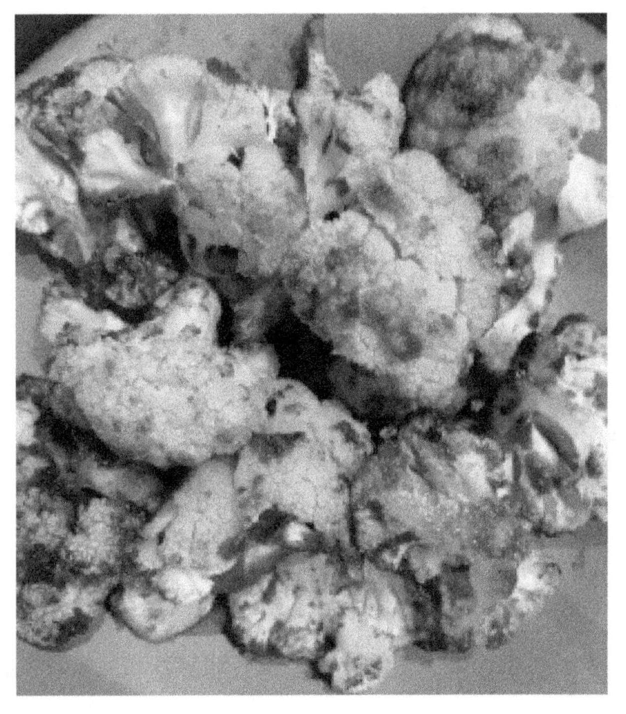

Total Time: 30 minutes

Difficulty Level: low

Servings: 5 Dozen

Ingredients:

- 1/2 cup of softened butter

- 1/2 cup of corn oil

- Four teaspoons of baking powder

- 1/2 cup of orange juice

- 1/2 cup of superfine sugar

- 1/2 cup of honey

- One teaspoon of ground cloves

- 1 1/2 cups of semolina

- Two teaspoons of lemon juice

- 1 cup of water

- *One orange, grated zest*

- *One cinnamon stick*

- *2 1/2 cups of all-purpose flour*

- *1/2 cup of finely chopped walnuts*

- *One teaspoon of ground cinnamon*

- *1 cup of white sugar*

Instructions:

Preheat oven to 350°F. A cookie sheet was oiled.

In a large mixing bowl, mix the orange zest, butter and superfine sugar. Incorporate the oil gradually and continue beating till smooth and creamy. Mix the flour, baking powder, cinnamon, semolina, and cloves; Alternately, add the orange juice to the fluffy mixture. As the mixture gets richer, transfer to a floured surface, kneading into a solid dough, with your fingers, shape tablespoonfuls of dough into balls or ovals. Arrange cookies two inches apart on prepared cookie sheets.

Bake for twenty minutes or till golden in a preheated oven. Allow baking sheets to cool completely before removing.

prepare the syrup:

In a medium-sized saucepan over medium heat, combine the cinnamon stick, water, honey, white sugar, and lemon juice.

Bring everything to a simmer, then reduce to low heat and continue cooking for 5 minutes.

Remove the cinnamon stick from the saucepan and set it aside.

Carefully dunk the cookies one by one into the boiling hot sauce, coating them completely.

Scatter walnuts over the top and set them aside to dry on a wire rack.

Position a scrap of paper beneath the rack to catch any drips.

Store the finished cookies in an airtight jar at room temperature.

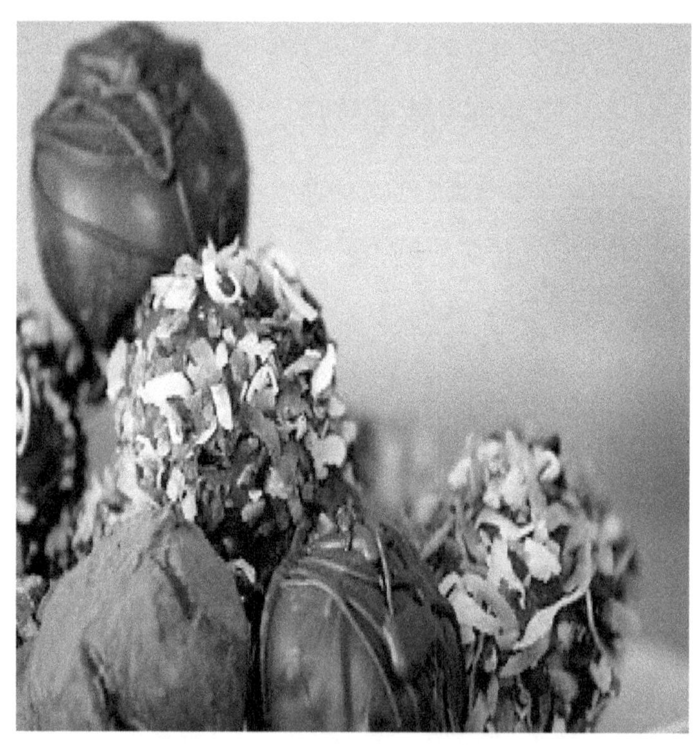

Total Time: 4 hours 20 minutes

Difficulty Level: low

Servings: 10

Ingredients:

- 2/3 cup sugar

- 2 tablespoons hot water

- 3 squares chopped semisweet chocolate

- Fresh mint leaves

- 1 tablespoon espresso powder or instant coffee granules

- 4 eggs, separated

- 1 teaspoon vanilla

- 3 tablespoons unsweetened cocoa powder, sifted

- Half teaspoon salt

- 2 egg whites

- Fresh raspberries

- 3 tablespoons margarine

- Thawed zero fat whipped topping

Instructions:

Preheat oven to 300° Fahrenheit (180 degrees Celsius). Preheat oven to 350 degrees Fahrenheit. Line the bottom of a greased 9-inch springform pan with parchment paper.

Melt the chocolate and margarine in a small heavy saucepan over low heat, constantly stirring, until smooth; leave aside to cool. Whisk together espresso powder and boiling water in a small cup. Whisk together six egg whites in a large mixing bowl and put them aside. In a medium mixing bowl, beat egg yolks on high speed for approximately 5 minutes or until pale yellow.

Add one-third cup sugar and beat for approximately 4 minutes, or until mixture, ribbons fall from the beaters. Beat in the melted chocolate mixture and espresso mixture on a low speed until barely blended, only before mixing the chocolate powder and vanilla extract.

Beat the egg whites on high speed for 2 minutes or add salt to taste until soft peaks form. Whisk together the remaining 1/3 cup sugar and the remaining white half of the egg in a separate bowl until firm. Stir a large scoop of egg whites into the chocolate mixture. Incorporate the chocolate mixture into the egg whites until almost completely combined. Pour the batter into the prepared pan.

Bake for 1 hour or until the cake begins to separate from the edges of the pan. Allow cooling on a wire rack for 10 minutes before running a thin spatula along the cake's perimeter. Remove the pan's sides one at a time, taking care not to scratch it. Allow for complete cooling before using. Invert the cake and cut away the bottom of the pan and the paper. After covering, refrigerate for a minimum of 4 hours. Garnish with whipped topping, raspberries, and mint, if preferred.

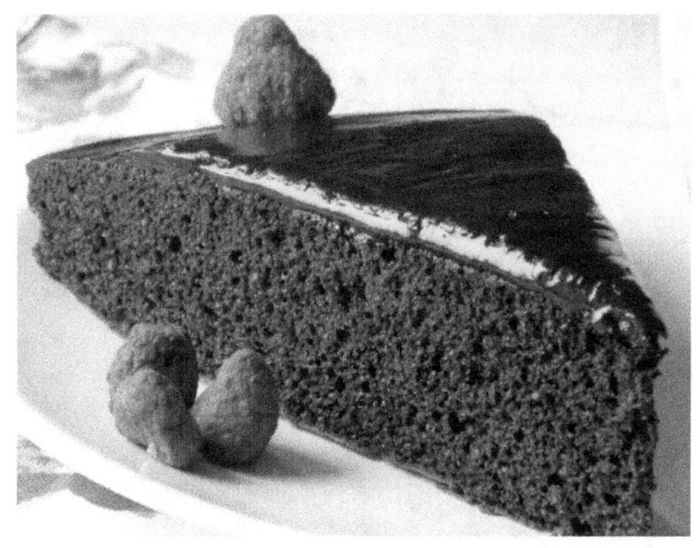

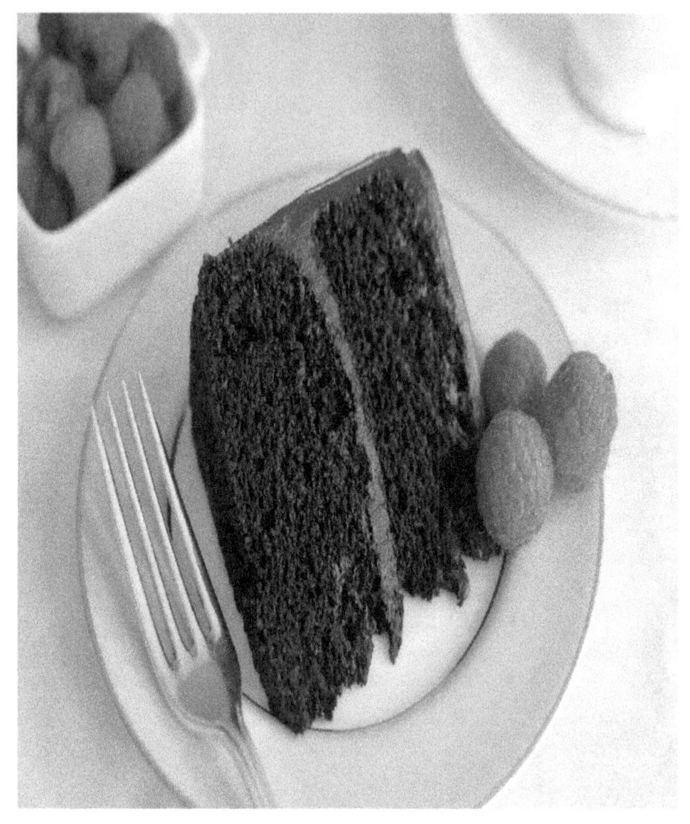

Total Time: 30 minutes

Difficulty Level: low

Servings: 15

Ingredients:

- *One package of cake mix lemon-flavored*

- *1/2 cup of canola oil*

- *One package of instant vanilla-flavored pudding mix*

- *1 cup of water*

- *Four medium-sized eggs, at the room temperature*

- *1/4 cup of poppy seeds*

For the drizzle/glaze:

- *Two tablespoons of fresh lemon juice*

- *2 cups of the confectioners' sugar*

- *Two tablespoons of water*

Instructions:

Preheat oven to 350°F.

In a large mixing bowl, add the eggs, pudding mix, oil, cake mix, and water and mix with an electric mixer on low speed for approximately 1 minute. Beat the butter at a medium speed for approximately 2 minutes. Combine the batter with the poppy seeds and transfer them into a prepared and dusted 13x9-inch baking dish.

Bake in the oven for approximately 20 to 25 minutes. After baking, transfer to a cooling rack.

Combine the lemon juice and confectioner's sugar and water in a small cup; drizzle over the cake and serve.

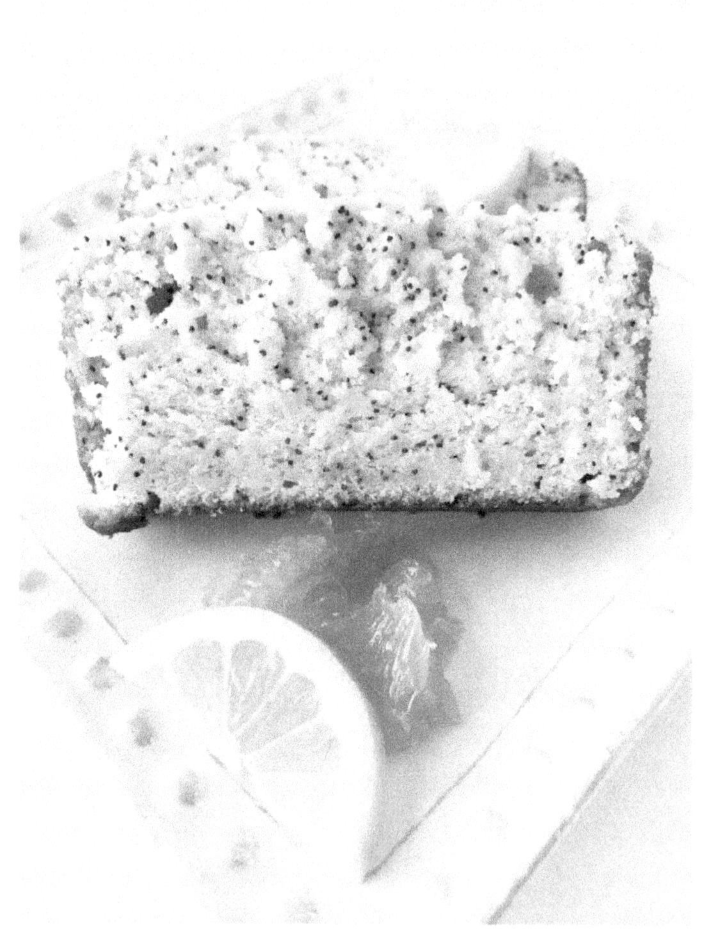

Total Time: 20 minutes

Difficulty Level: low

Servings: 4 Dozen

Ingredients:

- 2 1/4 cups of all-purpose flour

- One large egg

- 1/2 teaspoon of vanilla extract

- 1 cup of softened butter

- 1/2 cup of confectioners' sugar for coating

- 1/2 teaspoon of almond extract

- 3/4 cup of white sugar

Instructions:

Preheat oven to 400°F. Oil a cookie sheet.

In a medium-sized mixing basin, cream together the butter, sugar, and egg until smooth. Mix the vanilla and almond extracts in a small mixing bowl. Combine the flour and water to form a dough. You may need to mix the batter by hand. At a time, form a tsp of cookie dough into balls, logs, or 'S' shapes. Arrange biscuits one to 1 inch apart on prepared cookie sheets.

Bake for approximately 10 minutes, or until golden and robust, in a preheated oven. Allow the cookies to cool completely before dusting with confectioners' sugar.

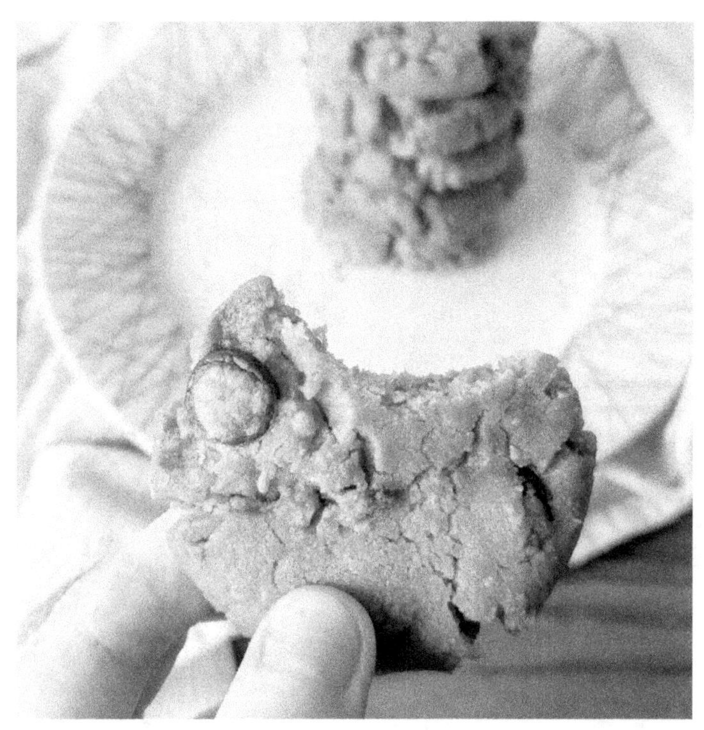

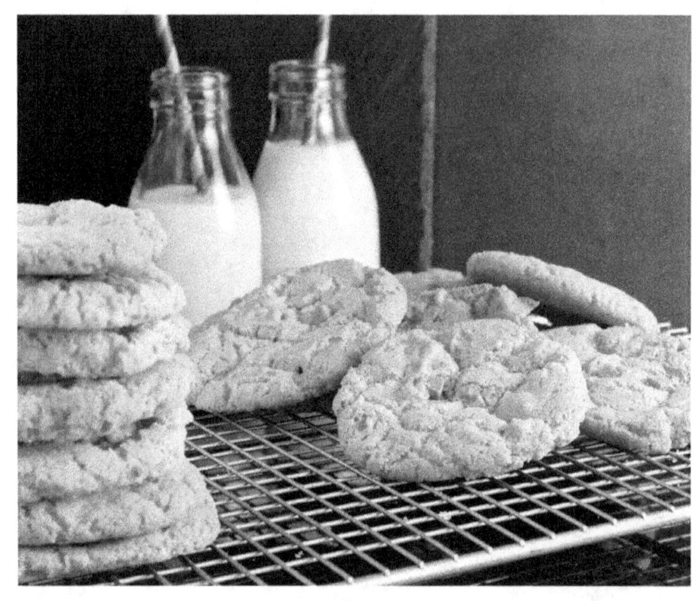

Total Time: 5 minutes

Difficulty Level: low

Servings: 2

Ingredients

- Greek yogurt, 1 cup

- Chocolate-hazelnut spread, ⅓ cup

- Almond butter, ½ cup

- Honey, one tablespoon

- Sliced fresh fruit

- Vanilla, one teaspoon

Instructions

To create a lighter, smoother dip, add all ingredients in a food processor; pulse until smooth.

Accompany with fresh berries.

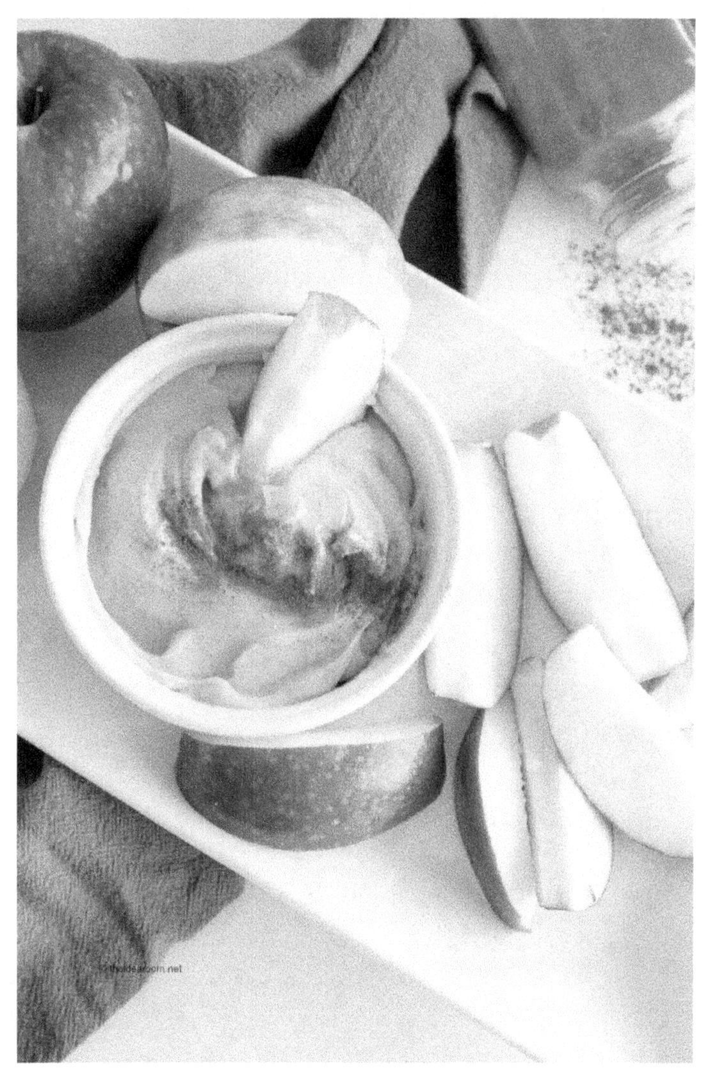

Total Time: 10 minutes

Difficulty Level: low

Servings: 4

Ingredients

- Pure peppermint extract, 1/8 teaspoon

- frozen bananas, 2

- natural food coloring

- Chocolate chips, 2-3 tablespoon

- Coconut cream, 1/2 cup

Instructions

Combine all of the ingredients in a mixing bowl and blend thoroughly with a hand mixer, then pour the mixture into a mold of your choice and freeze for up to 5-6 hours, then remove and scoop out the required quantity for serving, garnishing with chocolate chips.

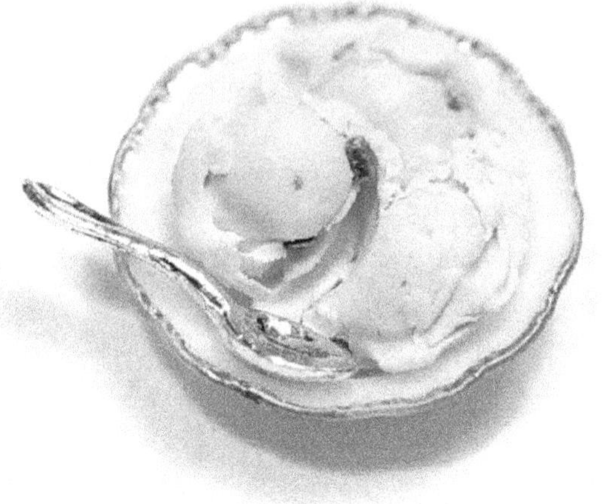

26. Rosé-Poached Peaches

Total Time: 15 minutes

Difficulty Level: low

Servings: 4

Ingredients

- Sugar, one tablespoon

- Fresh peaches, 1-pound

- Rose wine, ½ cup

- Green peppercorns, one teaspoon

Instructions

Mix the honey, rose, and peppercorns in a medium-sized pot. Bring to a simmer and then remove from the heat.

Cook for 5 minutes, uncovered. Gently fold in the peaches. Bring the water to a gentle simmer.

Cook, uncovered, for 1 minute. Transfer the mixture to a medium mixing cup. Refrigerate for three days.

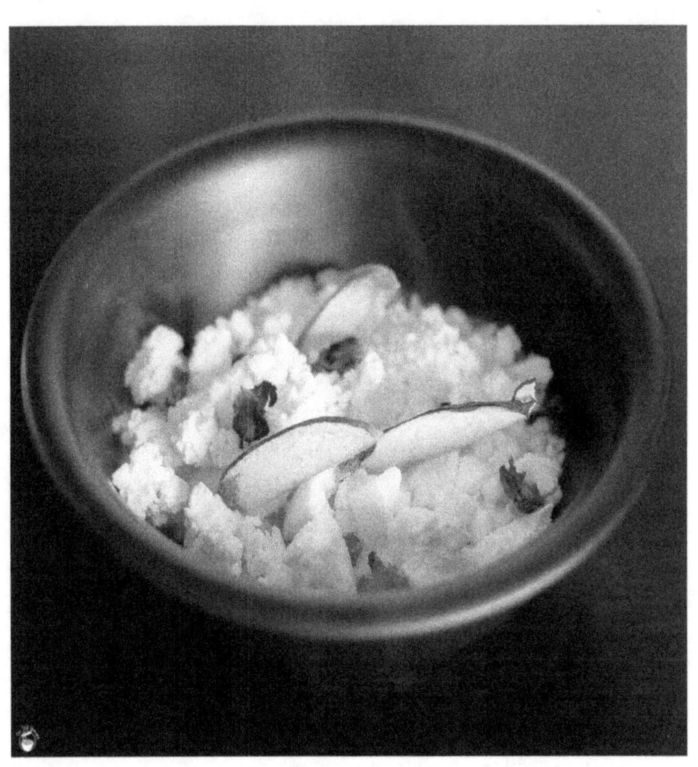

Total Time: 30 minutes

Difficulty Level: low

Servings: 2

Ingredients

- Cooked Ladyfingers, 3 ounces

- Brewed espresso, ¼ cup

- Carton mascarpone cheese, 8 ounces

- Whipping cream, 1 cup

- Powdered sugar, ¼ cup

- Vanilla, one teaspoon

- Chocolate liqueur, ⅓ cup

- White chocolate, 1 ounce

- Bittersweet chocolate, grated, 1 ounce

- Unsweetened cocoa powder

Instructions

Ladyfingers should be used to line the bottom of an 8x8x2-inch baking pan, trimmed to fit. Mix mascarpone, cheese, and whipping cream in a mixing bowl, along with powdered sugar and vanilla extract, until stiff peaks form.

Combine the chocolate liqueur and then evenly distribute half of the mascarpone mixture over the ladyfingers.

Finally, combine the mascarpone mixture and bittersweet chocolate. On top, add a layer of ladyfingers. Keep layering with the remainder of the espresso and mascarpone cheese. Refrigerate for approximately 8–16 hours.

The chocolate powder can be sprinkled on the dessert. If desired, garnish with cocoa beans.

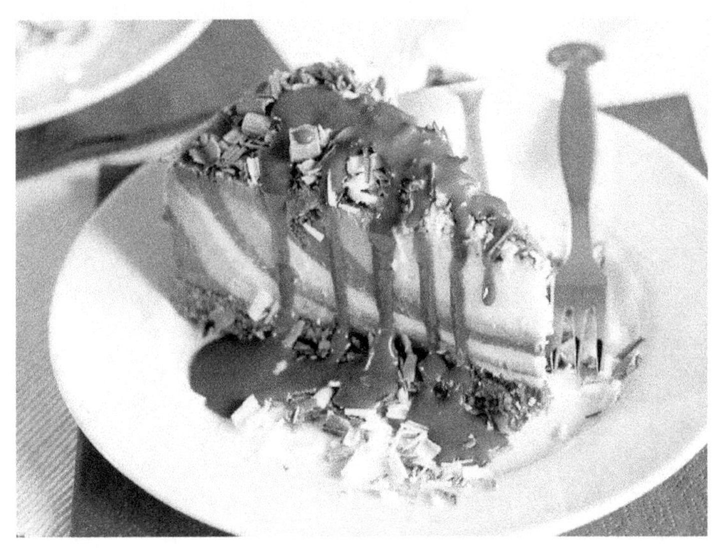

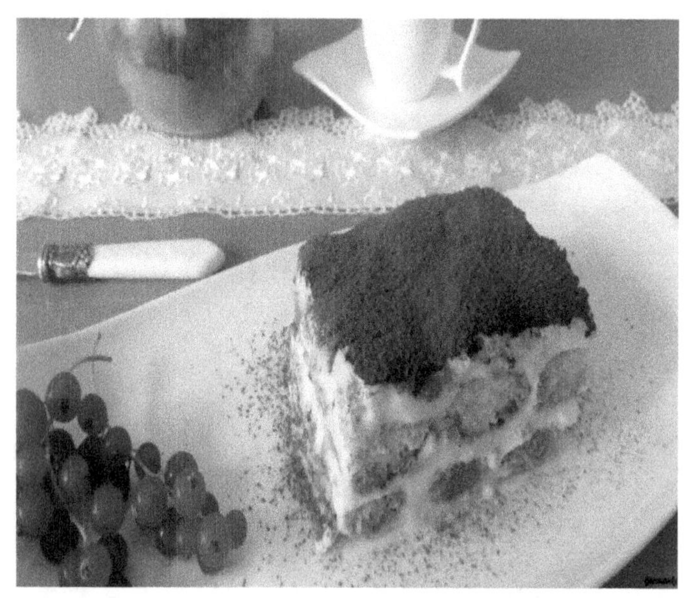

Total Time: 1 hour

Difficulty Level: low

Servings: 7

Ingredients:

- 1 cup smooth peanut butter
- 2/3 cup erythritol
- Half tsp vanilla essence
- Half tsp baking soda
- 1 large egg

Instructions:

Preheat oven to 350°F (180°C) and line a baking sheet with parchment paper. Take the item out of circulation.

Using a Nutribullet or a blender, powder the erythritol. Take the item out of circulation. This step can be omitted if a confectioner's low-carb sweetener is used.

In a medium mixing bowl, whisk together all ingredients until a smooth, glossy dough forms.

Roll two teaspoons of dough between your palms to form a ball and set it on the prepared cookie pan. Continue until the dough is depleted. This recipe should yield 12-14 cookies.

Using a fork, flatten the cookies, creating a crisscross pattern over the end.

Preheat oven to 350 degrees Fahrenheit and bake the cookies for 12–15 minutes.

Remove from the oven and cool for 25 minutes on the baking pan before transferring to a cooling rack to cool for an additional 15 minutes.

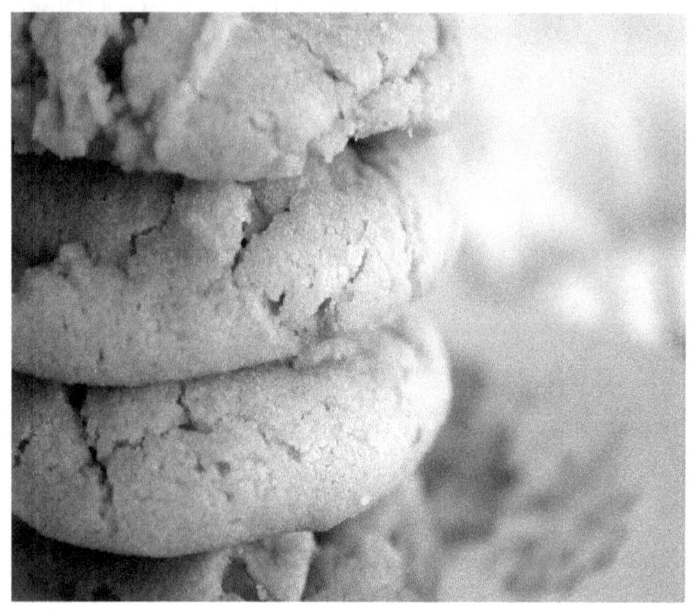

Total Time: 10 minutes

Difficulty Level: low

Servings: 3

Ingredients

- Oranges, 4

- the ground cinnamon, one tablespoon

- Raw Pistachios, 35g

- Extra-virgin olive oil one teaspoon

Instructions:

After washing the oranges and removing the skin, thinly slice them with a knife; chop the pistachios and scatter them over the orange slices at the end; drizzle with extra-

virgin olive oil and sprinkle with cinnamon;
serve.

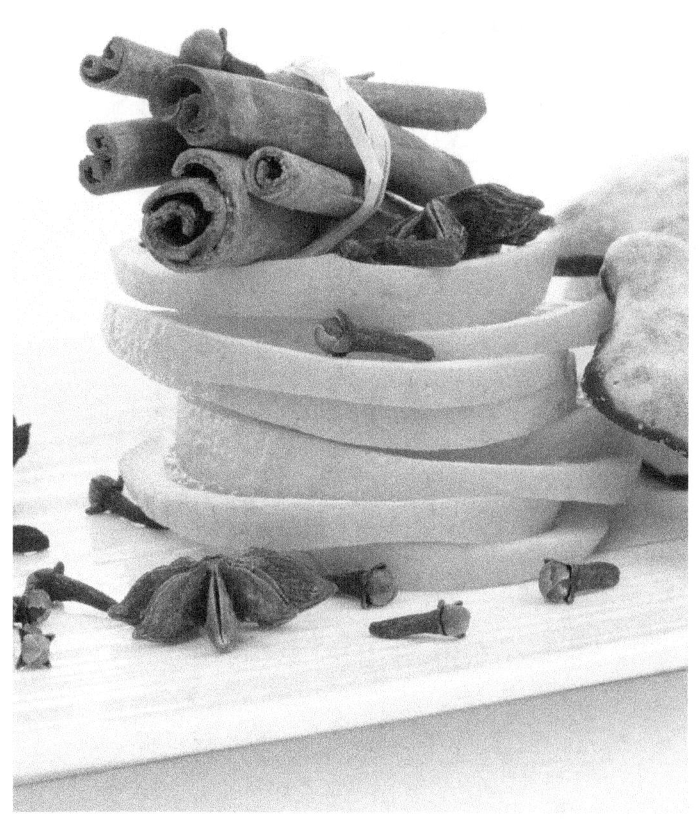

Total Time: 15 minutes

Difficulty Level: low

Servings: 4

Ingredients

- Creamy Peanut Butter, 1/2 cup

- Old Fashioned Oats, 1 cup

- Ground Flax Seeds, 1/4 cup

- Pure Maple Syrup, three tablespoons

- Dried Dates Pitted, 3 Oz

- Cinnamon, ground, 1/2 teaspoon

- Sea Salt, 1/4 teaspoon

- Pure Vanilla Extract, 1 1/2 teaspoon

- Chopped Pecans, 1/2 cup

Instructions

Mix the peanut butter and oats with vanilla extract and pitted dates in a food processor. Add the flax seeds, maple syrup, cinnamon, and a touch of salt. Now, combine the ingredients vigorously until smooth.

Pulse multiple times throughout the procedure to evenly distribute the pecans throughout the mixture.

Shape the mixture into little balls; approximately 2 tsp of the mixture will yield one ball. Now place these balls in an airtight jar and refrigerate; these balls will keep for up to 7 days if stored in the refrigerator.

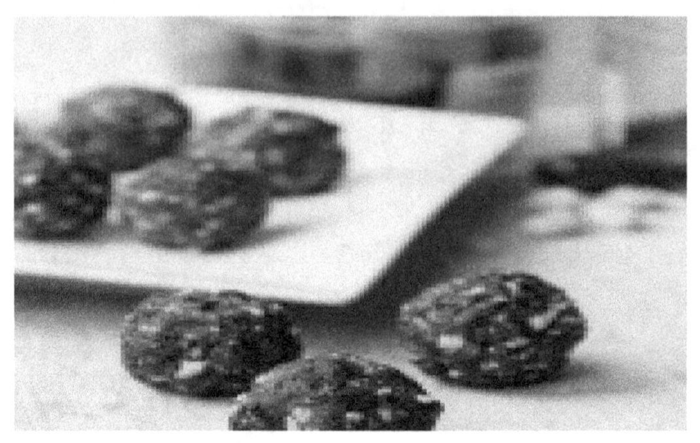

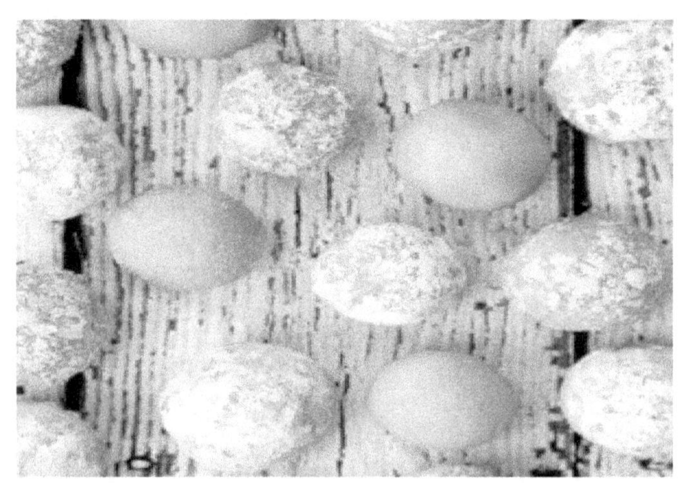

9 781803 612881